Kimberly D'Erar

10 Tips to Thriving

A Doctor's Guide to Accessing Full Vitality

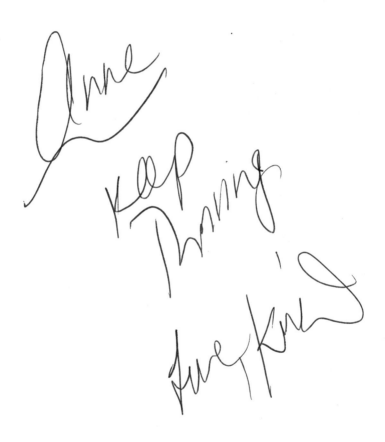

Anne,

Keep Thriving

Kim Kim

Disclaimer Regarding Expectations of Results – Dr. Kim D'Eramo and the publisher accept no liability for the use or misuse of the information contained in this book. There is no possibility of substantiating any claimed results made or supplying any objective evidence, whether financial, business related, spiritual or otherwise. Dr. Kim D'Eramo and the publisher strongly advise that you seek professional advice as appropriate before making any health decision. It can be assumed that no results are to be expected as a result of one's purchase of this book. Dr. Kim D'Eramo and the publisher do not and cannot make any representations, promises or guarantees of the effectiveness of this book. That being said, Dr. Kim D'Eramo and her associates, partners and affiliates firmly believe in the effectiveness of the methods put forth in this book.

Published by Global Medical Innovations, LLC.
PO Box 257
Woburn, MA
01801 USA

Visit our website: http://thethrivedoctors.com
Please send errors to info@thethrivedoctors.com

Technical Editor: Mario Torres-Leon, M.D.

ISBN 978-0-9890183-3-3
First Edition

Our true security and sense of worthiness comes not from our job, our kudos, our degrees or even our contribution to others.

True security is unwavering and stems from our own sense of self-acceptance and self-love.

This is created within and is available to us all.

Open with courage to receive this, and BE FULLY ALIVE.

This will change the world.

Acknowledgments

This book is my first, but it is the breakthrough I have needed in being brave enough to get my inner wisdom on paper. Many more are already being written, so this acknowledgment is really to thank all involved for my "great work."

Thank you so dearly to The Universe for being on my side, always being there for me and bringing me through every challenge in my life to meet this moment! I am immensely grateful for having created this book and brought it to fruition.

Thank you to our amazing Thrive Doctors support team: Keith Heustis, for your amazing patience and diligence in creating all of our work; Teresa Marks for literally bringing me into the next evolution of myself; and to Chris Gilbert for capturing it on film. Thank you all for believing in us every step of the way and being so committed to our vision.

Thank you to all of my mentors: Jane Carriero, D.O. and Donald Hankinson, D.O., for teaching me how to be a great osteopath; Greg Thompson, D.O., for all of your wisdom and getting me through residency without medication; Christiane Northrup, M.D. for your courage in paving the way and for telling me I could do it too.

Thank you to Joan Borysenko, M.D. and Larry Dossey, M.D. for your courageous and expansive work in the field of medicine. To Esther Hicks for your infinite wisdom and service. To Dr. Joe Vitale for your outlandish willingness to tell the truth. Thank you to Nancy Risley for RYSE; discovering your work connected me to myself in a way that nothing else did. Thank you to Shiva Rea and Beryl Bender Birch for your immense yogini wisdom; working with you was deeply inspiring in every moment. Thank you to Regina Thomashauer for giving me so much permission to be absolutely whatever I am.

Thank you to all of my patients. I heard your call all the way back in residency and it is what brought me through. Serving you has been an immense honor and something that has grown me every day.

Thank you to Apollonia Fortuna for teaching me how to listen and be present. This, of all the things I have learned, is the skill that has most helped me to serve.

Thank you to Paul Czeck for showing me your "B's," believing in me, and being one of the greatest friends I have ever had. Thank you to my "Providence College girls" for believing in me, being there for me, and always bringing me back to who I am. Thank you to Andrea Perella for being able to understand me no matter what I may say, and always make it matter.

Thank you to my godfather, Carmine, for shedding a tear every time I cross a finish line, and to all of my aunts, uncles, my niece, nephews and cousins. Thank you to my sister for being my cheerleader, and my brother for your support in coming to see me speak.

Thank you to my parents: my father for making me strong, and my mother for showing me what to do with it. You are the ones who deserve to celebrate my every success.

Thank you to my incredible husband, Mario. You mean more to me than anything in the world and you are my living proof every single day that my dreams are meant to come true. Marrying you and having our daughter are the things I am most proud of in my life. I may never understand the challenge I went through to get here, but it has awakened me to serve the world in a bigger way. Thank you for being on this journey with me.

Table of Contents

Introduction

Doctors are taught to treat illness and reverse disease, and conventional medicine is excellent at preventing death and prolonging life. However, for a majority of patients, much is lacking in the current medical model. So many patients have come to me in the emergency room and in my osteopathic practice struggling with pain, depression or some form of chronic illness. There are a vast amount of medications I have given to treat these symptoms, but, for the majority of these patients, medications did not address the source of their illness was not addressed.

Many patients are underserved when it comes to conventional medicine. These patients desire more than just living longer or having to rely on medication with harmful side effects. They want to feel vibrancy and vitality, passion and exuberance throughout their body. They also want to consistently experience their highest level of inspiration and aliveness beyond their physical body through their relationships, career and in their outer life. This experience is what I call the **state of Thriving**.

While conventional medicine has many brilliant technologies, it has not really offered anything to help patients thrive. Medications can reverse symptoms, but they have limited value in connecting us with our Life Force, the source of healing within. When patients seeking to thrive look to their physicians, the doctor is often at a loss to offer something that has this impact, and may even tell the patient that it is not possible for them to feel this way. It isn't that doctors don't care deeply about their patients; it's just that many of them have not been taught about the modalities that are available to create this possibility.

As an osteopathic physician, I was taught to understand and appreciate that the source of healing lies within us. I would educate my patients about this, and treat them osteopathically to help open themselves to this source and remove any barriers to receiving it. My results were sometimes limited, however. There were patients who would get better for a time, only to return with the same problems again and again: depression, pain, and illness. I realized that although they would feel better physically, once they returned to their toxic relationships, toxic job situations and toxic ways of thinking, their physical vigor would eventually diminish. The ways they engaged in life limited their ability to really thrive. If I wanted to assist my patients in making real changes in their health, I needed to assist them in making real changes in their life. I needed to help them change the way they think and relate.

This desire revolutionized the approach I took in my career. I created an intensive course designed to educate patients about the state of Thriving that is available to us all. In this course, I teach that it is our thoughts and beliefs that either open us to the Life Force or limit our experience of it. Even the way we respond to medication and medical procedures is dependent upon our thoughts and beliefs. Our ability to experience this Life Force within creates healthy, vibrant cells; healthy, vibrant emotions; and a healthy, vibrant life – or the lack thereof.

I wrote this book to give you an introduction in connecting with your Life Force and to provide some easy tips that will help you begin to experience it in ever-greater amounts. My intention is that we each individually embrace this within ourselves and create a world of thriving.

I invite you to visit our website and download your free MP3 audio: "The Universal Principles of Thriving." Go to: www. thethrivedoctors.com/gift for your free audio gift!

We also have information on our products and live courses, as well as other free resources to assist you in Thriving! www.thethrivedoctors.com

Premise of this Book

When I was a child, my siblings and I would play a game where one of us would have to find something hidden. If I walked toward the item, the others would say, "You're getting hot!" If I walked in the wrong direction, they would say, "Cold." The closer I got to the item, the more they would yell: "HOT! Smoking! Steaming!" or "You're on fire!" to indicate that I was very, very close. When I was very close and turned away even slightly, they would indicate that I was cold or even freezing. The closer I got, the more precise my indicator would be.

As a living, breathing human being, your body is constantly communicating to you whether you are hot or cold, too. What you are moving toward or away from is your ideal state. This ideal state is the state of Thriving. It is your Truth. When you have thoughts that are counter to your Truth, your body and your life give you signals that you are cold. You don't feel well, you have low energy, things are difficult for you, and nothing goes your way. When you have thoughts that are in sync with your Truth, your body feels good. You have increased energy and vitality. Life also responds and things seem to work themselves out for you effortlessly.

As a physician, I am intimately familiar with the signals and communication pathways in the body. I understand the physiology behind our internal states. Throughout this book, I explain this physiology for you, so that you understand what is happening within your body and how your internal guidance system works. I offer the ten best lessons or tips that I use to stay in the state of Thriving. I share some of my favorite quotes, and answer the most common questions that come up for my patients and in my courses regarding each tip. Each chapter ends with a tool for you to use to integrate this tip into your life, and an affirmation or meditation to complete the process.

The Biochemistry of Thriving

What is thriving? Thriving is the experience of your highest vision of vitality and aliveness in all areas of life. It's that feeling of being turned on and fully alive. Thriving is that state of completion and fulfillment for which we are all longing. It is your natural state and it is your birthright.

You do not need to be someone special or accomplish something significant to experience thriving. Thriving happens when you are aligned with your life's purpose and highest level of self-expression. You thrive when you live as who you authentically are. You can connect with this state at any time from whatever state you are in. Thriving is actually available to you right now!

How you think about yourself and your life has a lot to do with whether you experience life in a state of Thriving or you don't. Your mind is actually in charge of all of your experiences. Every thought you have is a biochemical reaction in your body, and these reactions have either positive or negative effects. Your thoughts affect every cell in your body and also have an effect on how you feel. Your entire internal state actually begins with your thoughts. It is your internal state that drives all of your actions and behaviors and dictates every single thing you do.

When you have "negative" thoughts, thoughts that go against your natural state and against your Truth, you generate biochemicals that are damaging to your cells. Any thoughts that cause anxiety, fear, anger, or even frustration and irritability generate these "negative biochemicals." These stressful thoughts ignite the fight-or-flight response in the body. Cortisol, epinephrine and norepinephrine, and the inflammatory cascade kick in and have an effect on all of your cells. These stress chemicals assist you in the short term, fueling the muscles, focusing the brain, increasing blood pressure and heart rate and making the heart pump more powerfully. The problem occurs when these hormones and stress chemicals are around for extended periods of time. Over time, these effects are harmful and cause cells to break down. The body is not designed to withstand chronic exposure to these biochemicals. However, for people living in intense states of anxiety and tension, these hormones stick around for much longer than intended and wreak havoc on the body. The heart is overworked, the increased blood pressure causes vascular damage, and the body's organs are impaired. We see these effects throughout our culture: chronic illnesses like heart disease, diabetes, and cancer are now rampant.

During this stress state, these biochemicals shunt blood away from the brain and gut to fuel muscles, so you do not properly break down and absorb nutrients the way you need to. Since these chemicals inhibit insulin and assist us in using fast sources of energy, we are not able to break down fats and utilize slower energy sources. For short-term periods of stress or intensity, it is useful for our brain to be focused on one thing and think of nothing other than the task at hand; however, in this state we lose the ability to see the bigger picture. With chronic stress, the brain cannot process large amounts of information, and does not have the insight to create solutions.

Also during this stress state, the vessels that feed the organs constrict to shunt the blood to the working muscles. This deprives the organs and tissues of oxygen and nutrients. Cells deteriorate and build up toxic waste products. This negative biochemical state even affects your DNA and turns on the genes for diseases like diabetes, heart disease and cancer. *Your limiting "negative" thoughts destroy you at the level of your cells and your DNA.*

When you have positive thoughts, thoughts that are in sync with your natural state of thriving, this generates "positive biochemistry" that is nurturing to your cells. Endorphins and oxytocin make you feel good. Antioxidants repair damage in your DNA and reverse illness and ageing. The immune system is strengthened and you are resistant to pathogens like bacteria and viruses. Your serotonin and other hormones balance out and create harmony. You feel good because your brain works as it is meant to, seeing the big picture and easily processing information to come up with creative solutions to make your life work. Even your DNA is affected so that healthy genes that strengthen your system and protect against illness are turned on and the genes for disease are turned off. *Life-giving, "positive" thoughts protect and strengthen you at the level of your cells and DNA!*

Your Many Minds

Most people think of the mind being centered in the brain; and for decades, this has been the scientific and medical understanding. The brain was thought to govern activity for all the areas of the body, and be the sole producer of neurotransmitters, the hormones that deliver information to the entire nervous system. Extensive research by the Institute for Heart Math has now demonstrated that this is not true. There are networks of nerve cells or "thinking cells," located all over the body, and distributed around various organs. A large proportion of this neural meshwork is located in the area around the heart. These nerve networks around the heart respond to neurotransmitters in the same way the brain does. Interestingly, the nerves in the area of the heart send large amounts information and signals to the brain that control brain activity. In fact, there is more information from the heart going to the brain to control and modulate brain function than from the brain to control the heart. Therefore, research has shown that the heart has far more input and control over brain activity and function than previously thought.

The nerve activity around the level of the heart can be detected with equipment to have an impact not just inside the body, but also up to eight to ten feet away from the body. It creates a field of electromagnetic energy that changes depending on the emotional state of the person. This activity is either "concordant" or "discordant." The "concordant" activity harmonizes organ function: evening out the heart rate, heart and respiratory function, normalizing blood pressure, and instilling smooth respiratory function. The "discordant" activity causes erratic variability in the heart rate, irregularity in the breathing, and abnormal shifts in the blood pressure. The "concordant" activity is detected from the area around the heart when a person is experiencing harmonic emotions, such as love, joy, peace and appreciation. "Discordant" activity is detected from the area around the heart when a person is experiencing disharmonic emotional states like anger, fear, frustration or impatience. The more negative the emotional state, the more erratic and disharmonic is the physiologic activity detected in the vital signs. *Therefore, your emotional state is directly linked to the quality of physiologic activity in your body.*

Your Emotions: The Key to Your Every Thought

There are many thoughts going through the mind at any given time. It would be impossible to keep track of them all. The thoughts you are aware of are only the tip of the iceberg, since most of your thoughts are unconscious. However, you do have the ability to be internally aware of what is going on at all times. Your emotions are the key to this awareness. *Your emotional state is the reflection of the sum of all the thoughts you are having at any given time.*

You can become aware of your emotions by connecting within, to how you feel. This takes practice. For decades we have all been taught to use our left brain in processing information, being aware of what we think and how to figure things out. We have been trained to ignore our feelings because they were thought to be irrelevant. However, your emotions have immense value. They give you insight as to whether the way you are thinking is generating a positive or a negative response in your body. When your thinking generates a negative response, you have lower emotions: anger, anxiety, fear. When your thinking generates a positive response, you feel higher emotions: joy, love, inspiration or appreciation. It is through accessing your emotions at any given moment that you become aware of the impact of the thoughts and beliefs you are holding, and any choice you may be considering.

If you were to rely on left-brained, rational thinking alone in making choices, do you have any idea how much information you would need to process before you could make an informed decision? Let's say you are deciding on what college is best for your child. You think about the location, the quality of education, the safety, the price of tuition, and many other important factors. Even if you could solidly nail down which school had the best mix of all of these factors, you still could not know which would provide your child the best mix of friends, social support, inspirational experiences, and opportunities for his or her ideal career and life. How would you best make the choice then? You would base it on how you feel.

Even if you think you are the most rational person you know and you think everything through before making a choice, I would tell you that your emotions are still running the show. When you walk into a room, your emotions determine where you choose to sit. Someone smells funny to you or someone has looks that make you feel uncomfortable. This type of awareness is happening way below the level of your conscious mind – you think you just liked the seat in the middle.

Let's say you want to go to get fit and lose weight. You have all the best intentions to get to the gym but you're tired, or hungry or someone calls you on the phone, so you decide not to go. You think you chose not to go to the gym because it made more sense to take that call or eat dinner, but the reason you didn't go is because your emotional state prevented you from going. It is your emotions that are inspiring you or dragging you down. When you are emotionally aligned with a certain outcome, your emotions trigger reminders or motivation to bring it about. You remember that it's time for an appointment or time to eat. So you arrive at your destination on time, or you eat a meal. It is your emotional state that drives your every action or behavior.

You can use the awareness of your emotional state to make shifts in your thinking. When you are in a negative emotional state, your choices and decisions will create results that reflect that negative state back to you. This happens automatically, unless you become aware and shift your emotional state. Becoming aware gives you a choice. You can be reactive and function on autopilot, or you can choose to shift your emotional state first, before acting, speaking, or doing anything. It is that simple. It becomes that easy.

The next section of the book contains Ten Thrive Tips to use in consciously shifting your emotional state in any given moment. The more you practice them, the more ingrained they become until this way of being is your autopilot and you effortlessly create a life that reflects what you do want. Even with initial use, however, you will begin to see major shifts in the external reality you are experiencing. It is my intention that you keep an open mind in allowing your personal transformation, being willing to persist in using your mind as the brilliant and powerful creative tool that it really is.

I invite your questions and comments on our website: www.thethrivedoctors.com, where we have other resources to assist you in Thriving!

"Let a man radically alter
his thoughts, and he will
be astonished at the rapid
transformation it will effect
in the material conditions
of his life."

— James Allen

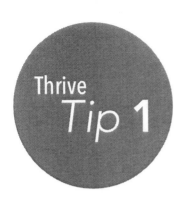

Thrive
Tip 1

Change Your Thoughts, Change Your Life

Are you working against yourself? If you are harboring negative thoughts or beliefs while doing things to get ahead and succeed in life, then the answer is a big, FAT, yes! So powerful are your thoughts that they can negate the benefits of even the best fitness routines and the healthiest of diets.

I can't count the number of patients I have seen who deeply want to be healthy and feel great, but who have not even begun to get to the root of why they are feeling depressed, carrying excess weight, or experiencing illness. Many toil away at the gym, take all kinds of supplements, do a cleanse, visit the doctor, all to no avail. If they do see results, they are hard- won and fleeting.

This happens because the root cause of imbalance and disease begins in your thoughts and beliefs. It won't matter what you do on the outside if your beliefs and thoughts are not aligned with what you are trying to achieve. It is your thoughts that create your internal conditions and your biochemistry. It is your thoughts that create your emotional state, which drives all of your actions and behaviors. If you want a change in your life, change your thoughts. When you change your mind you change your health; you change your life.

Yes, genetics plays a role. Yes, what you eat affects your health. Yes, exercise does make you feel great. But the impact of these is minor compared to the power of the millions of thoughts you are having in every moment. Even a person with a terrible genetic predisposition can exhibit perfect health when his thoughts are aligned with thriving.

How can you change your thoughts if you can't even know what most of them are? Since most of your thoughts are unconscious, you could hold the thought: "I'm a great success" and still feel like a total loser because of the quality of your unconscious thoughts. That is where accessing your emotions comes in. The only way you can truly change to more positive thoughts is by getting yourself into a higher emotional state.

How would it feel to be living your ideal life? How would you feel to be a massive success with plenty of money, a beautiful lover and a healthy, fit body? When you can get into that feeling and embrace it, let it wash over you and bathe your cells, *you actually attract the experience to you.*

You initiate the positive biochemical state by feeling your desired outcome. Endorphins and oxytocin – feel-good hormones – increase, hormonal balance occurs, oxidation and toxicity decrease, and you feel better. When you feel your desired outcome, the fight-or-flight response of the sympathetic nervous system gets turned off. Cortisol and stress hormones decrease and your body restores normal function. Inflammation decreases so your body is no longer reactive and irritated. The parasympathetic nervous system kicks in and allows physiologic balance. You absorb nutrients, excrete waste, and oxygenate your organs and tissues, When you get into the emotional state that matches your desired outcome, you begin to establish better health immediately, and you behave in ways that are consistent with Thriving because you feel great.

Also, since positive emotions harmonize the mind at the level of the heart, your physiology is balanced and the brain function improves. Have you ever been in a stressful experience and not been able to find the right words, and then find later when the situation is long over, the witty words that would have brought perfect resolution come to mind? That's because you are no longer in the stress state. When you are in the relaxation state, the right words come effortlessly and you have insight in how to perfectly handle situations.

When you are in this relaxation state, your proprioception is enhanced and you perform better at whatever you are doing. If you're a tennis player and you want to win, generating a positive emotional state by embracing positive thoughts will actually bring about enhanced performance. If you are nervous about a meeting or a date, conjuring up winning thoughts first and generating an emotional shift will enhance your ability to be yourself and get your point across. You end up with wins at work or harmony and fun on a date. Therefore, when you think you are a success, you find that you are.

The reason you can't override your thoughts and internal state is because they are communicated in everything you do. Ninety-three percent of what you communicate is in your body language, tone, volume, and pace, not in your content. These things cannot be faked. These are subconscious communications. They have an impact on everything around you.

Think of a nervous person, filled with fear and anxiety and having thoughts of "I'm a loser and everyone knows it." How would his voice sound if he were to say: "Respect me. I'm worth listening to!" Would you listen to this person and follow? Now think of that same person holding thoughts of power. He feels certain and confidant and says: "I am a massive success and can do anything I choose." He has fully embodied this empowered emotional state. Would you rely on this person and follow?

When you think winning thoughts and generate a matching emotional state, it comes across in your communication and you have impact and power. This affects your work and all of your relationships. That's why when you feel like you're worthless, others treat you as such. They can't not! They're receiving your unconscious communication, and it's more powerful than your words.

Your impact is directly related to your internal state. Everyone knows what is going on inside you even on a subconscious level, and they will respond and treat you accordingly. Your life will always reflect your thoughts about yourself. Choose thriving thoughts, and you create a thriving life. Feel the emotions of your desired outcome, and you generate thoughts and messages that match it.

Thrive Tool

Consider these empowering thoughts and tune into the way they make you feel.

"I am worthy of love and belonging."
"I am brilliant and valuable."
"I am healthy and filled with vitality."

Hold that feeling in your body for several breaths and receive it. Breathe this way until you feel an emotional shift inside.

Question

Isn't this unrealistic? How can I think these positive thoughts when I know they are not true?

There is a difference between your truth and the Real Truth. Your current experience is true and is real for you. It isn't necessarily the Real Truth, however. It's just your interpretation of reality. The Real Truth is that life responds to your beliefs, and you will always see evidence to support what you currently think. It actually takes willingness to consider a new possibility and to begin to embrace a different experience before you see evidence of that new belief. You are right that your experience is really happening and the limitations you have are really true for you. You can also let that go and embrace a new truth and choose to live it. You can be right or you can be happy. You choose.

Let the new thoughts in, even if they are not apparent in your reality. Begin to base your thoughts and beliefs not on what you are currently experiencing, but on what you would like to be true. Choose thoughts that make you feel how you would like to feel.

Question your beliefs. Find your most negative belief and ask: "Can I know for sure that this is actually true?" Do you know anyone for whom this new idea is true? Also, do you know instances where your old beliefs were not actually true? For example: "I need to work hard to have money." Do you know anyone who doesn't work hard and who has plenty of money? Do you know anyone who works very hard and still has no money? Begin to question your conclusions and create space for new ideas and beliefs.

Affirmation

"I stay in a state of ease and grace, and life reflects this back to me."

"Be still and know that I am God."

— Psalm 46:10

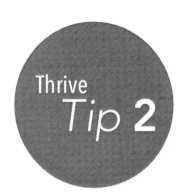

Thrive *Tip* **2**

A, B, C (Awaken, Breathe, Choose)

How often have you begun your day and known it was or was not going to be a "good" day? How often have you felt subject to external circumstances that seemed to dictate whether your day would or would not go well?

Does it feel sometimes like your entire life is subject to random chance that dictates whether or not things will turn out the way you want them to? It's time to wake up!

Your life is entirely within your own control and ability to make what you want it to be. You just haven't learned where the controls are. Maybe you never even realized that you are actually the one in control. No wonder life has not turned out the way you want it to. So forgive yourself for what you have created thus far. Let go of the past, and get in the driver's seat. I'm going to show you how to use some of the controls.

Your thoughts affect every cell in your body. They generate the biochemical state that sets the stage for everything that happens in your body and they set your emotional state. Your thoughts also create. On a quantum level, reality is made of all the same stuff, and this stuff is energy. Your thoughts have an energetic impact on everything around you and things remote. Most of your thoughts are unconscious, they're pre-programmed and run on autopilot creating the same things over and over again. You don't need to understand biochemistry or physics to put the particles of matter together and create; your energetic system is creating your life for you. The reality you are currently creating will match the emotional state you are in now. So get a handle on where you are right now. From there, all you need to do is bring yourself to a better emotional state, which develops better-feeling thoughts. Since your thoughts create your life, you develop a better life!

How do you raise your emotional state? I've come up with a way you can use in any given moment: A, B, C.

A. Awaken

Become aware of how you are feeling right now. Do this on a scale of 0–10, ten being the best. Rate your emotional level and acknowledge it.

Your awareness of your internal state actually shifts your biochemistry immediately. This shift occurs because it changes the thoughts you are having. You shift from having unconscious thoughts, which are

...ing, to being consciously
your internal state. Typically
u are struggling, hurting, or
cing something that you do not
ecomes so severe it wakes you up.
ing, although it may not feel so great.
Someth... ie pain and discomfort may get so bad,
you find yourself on your knees asking for another way.
It doesn't matter how bad you feel, what matters is
that you awaken. Become aware of how you feel.

Most people live in an unawakened state. In this state,
the subconscious programming runs the show for
your life. The subconscious is your default mode, and
studies show that more than 70% of our unconscious
thoughts are negative. Until you align it with the
beliefs you want, life will not be fulfilling. You can
live in default mode, only becoming aware at the
point of suffering, or you can choose to consciously
awaken at any time. Do this simply by focusing on your
internal state. This happens in the present moment.
Your internal state is never something in the past or
something in the future. Therefore, becoming aware
this way anchors you in the *now*, where all things
occur.

B. Breathe

Take three deep, present, mindful breaths. The breath actually has the ability to transform your biochemical and energetic state immediately. When you slow your breath down, you change from the fight-or-flight style breathing to the relaxation breathing, which generates the positive biochemical state. This turns off the sympathetic nervous system, (stress response, cortisol, epinephrine, inflammation, limited ability to process new information) and turns on the parasympathetic nervous system (hormonal balance, oxytocin, endorphins, restoration of energy.) Breathing this way shifts the neuronal activity in the brain and actually changes the information that the brain is registering. Areas of the brain that store positive thoughts are activated and positive thoughts are triggered. This type of breathing gives you an expanded perspective and ability to process information, and makes you feel better immediately.

C. Choose

From this expanded and aware state, after slowing things down with the breath, you are able to choose your action. Choose what feels right to you. You probably have an idea of some choices that are appropriate to thrive in life: choosing to exercise, choosing to eat real foods, choosing to be compassionate with others, choosing to treat yourself with kindness, etc. When you're in a stress state, however, you don't make these choices easily. You have food cravings and grab whatever's available. You criticize others and speak harshly. You feel sluggish and sit around instead of going for a walk. Most of the time you are reacting to your external situations. You haven't been able to make the choice to thrive, because when things are coming at you so fast, you can't even see the options. When you wake up and shift your internal state by using your breath to slow things down, you feel better and you make better choices. These choices are the habits for your thriving life.

Thrive Tool

Allow your abdomen to relax and take in slow, deep, present breaths while you allow whatever is going on to just be. Watch your internal state by focusing your attention on it. Allow it to just be without following the impulse to do anything.

Hold that feeling in your body for several breaths and receive it. Breathe this way until you feel an emotional shift inside.

Question

How can I stop when something really needs my attention? I have to react quickly or it will not be okay.

No matter what you are doing, you must breathe. As an ER doctor, I have been in life or death situations many times. Nowhere in my life has it been so apparent the importance of breathing and slowing things down. When I was stressed and couldn't think straight, it was impossible to recall the myriad of medications and algorithms I needed to access. Whenever I got present and breathed mindfully, the things I did had the impact I wanted them to have. Getting present like this gave me access to everything from calculating the correct drug dosage to performing life-saving procedures. When you slow down and breathe this way, you can use your mind as the brilliant machine it really is. Trust this and let it work for you. It changes everything and makes life work.

Meditation

Let whatever is bothering you leave with the exhaled breath. Just exhale it out. See this old energy leaving you. Bring in peace and love as you inhale. See your body fill up with light as you receive each breath.

Do this several times a day and any time you would like to feel free, secure, or clear-headed.

"Problems cannot be solved with the same mindset that created them."

— *Albert Einstein*

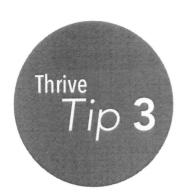

Thrive
Tip 3

Focus on what You DO Want

You may think about an issue you are dealing with and complain to a friend, obsess in fear that nothing will get better, or ruminate over why something negative is happening to you. It's typical to focus on what you don't want, because things that are bothersome get your attention. As a doctor, people come to me to address their problems and complaints. They tend to focus on what's wrong. Doctors have been trained to focus on the symptom or disease, and patients are accustomed to think in terms of problems. This happens not only in medicine, but in every area of life. Even when people talk about what they do want, it's framed in terms of what they do not want: "I hope I don't get sick," "I don't want to go into debt." "I want to get out of this pain." "I don't want to date any more losers."

It's time to retrain your brain. What you focus on expands. Whatever you put your mind on creates your internal state. When you focus your attention on what you DO want it feels good. Why? There are several reasons. When you bring your attention to what you do want, you immediately begin to generate the positive biochemicals that nourish your cells and create a higher emotional state. Oxytocin and endorphins block pain receptors and stimulate the receptors for pleasure, so you get relief from focusing on your pain or discontent. You feel better, and when you feel better it's easier to focus on the positive side of things. In the positive biochemical state, the mind is able to process information more easily and opens to new insights and creative solutions you previously could not see. Since the mind is able to see the big picture, you can see beyond the problem, making it easier to keep your focus on what you DO want.

Here is the most interesting part: focusing on what you do want also changes the hardwiring of your brain. The neurons in the brain connect to other neurons at junctions called synapses. These neural synapses are constructed in a certain pattern, so the same information gets transmitted over and over along these pathways. That makes it easy for you to keep thinking the same thoughts over and over without even trying. However, the brain has "neuroplasticity," which is the ability to change its wiring, construct new pathways and alter the old pathways. When you change your focus, you actually change the way information is handled in the brain and you make new pathways to carry this new information.

If you are of a negative mindset, your current neural wiring is not able to carry very high frequency positive thoughts. This is why new thoughts like "I am amazing and life is perfect just as it is" get bumped out of the system! You cannot carry information that is dramatically different from what you are currently thinking and believing. You need to alter your wiring first so that highly positive thoughts will stick and your mind will transmit the information. Your mind will not accept information it cannot neurologically integrate. You need to create new neurological pathways that can hold this new type of information. You do this by focusing your attention on what you do want.

The more you practice this, the more aware you become of the things that please you, so they suddenly seem to be more abundant. Receptors in the brain shift and adjust and your neural pathways become more adept at letting this type of information in. You begin to notice this new information everywhere because you have literally changed the information your brain can receive. Therefore, you enhance your brain's capacity to carry this positive information the more you focus on what you DO want.

Bring your mind's attention to things that please you. This can be anything: joy over your child, awe at the sunset, that cool pair of shoes you look so cute in, or living the life of your dreams. The brain does not know the difference between actual vs. imagined reality.

It will generate positive chemicals whether you are experiencing something you love or just thinking about it, and it will generate negative chemicals when you think about something you do not want.

Thrive Tool

Anytime you find yourself unhappy, complaining, or experiencing anything you do not want, turn it around to its opposite and be aware of what you DO want. Just flip it! If you notice you might be late, think "I want to be on time." If you notice you're feeling fatigued, think "I want to feel vibrant and alert."

If you find yourself complaining to a friend: "He's always late." Turn this to: "I want him to pick me up on time." Find all the ways you have been training your brain to be negative and turn them around!

Question

I'm thinking positive thoughts and nothing's happening. Why isn't this working for me?

The chemical shifts happen immediately, and before long the positive chemicals will outweigh the negative ones and you will have an emotional shift. However, the neural pathways in the brain take time before they rewire. That means you have to be persistent with this practice. Once you have shifted emotionally, you are in the positive biochemical state and your brain has an increased capacity to consider new ideas and beliefs. This is when new ideas will stick and you will be able to hold them. The brain then begins to handle this new information and changes in the hardwiring occur.

Affirmation

"I am powerful and create whatever I think about."

"Whether a man believes he can or he cannot, he is always right."

— *Henry Ford*

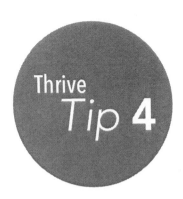

Thrive
Tip 4

Use Your Words

Your words are one of the most powerful creative forces you use every day. By now you understand that your thoughts affect your cells, your emotions, and all of your experiences, yet your words are even more powerful than your thoughts, because instead of just floating around in your head, they are concrete manifestations you put out into the world. *Your words are the beliefs you hold most strongly.*

When words are spoken, whether they are true or not, your brain begins to process the information as if it were true, that's why some forms of advertising can be so powerful. Your brain absorbs the nice woman on the commercial as if she were your trusted friend. She looks like your trusted friend and sounds like a reliable person, so the information is absorbed by the brain and is accepted. This information can be about anything from the value of a hair product to the certainty of your financial demise. If the words you speak cause fear, you create an immediate negative biochemical response. This destroys you at the level of your cells and DNA and so creates the reality that you are afraid of.

The reason the words someone says are integrated and accepted is because, on some level, you respect the person speaking them, or have in some way given power to that person. That's why when your mother tells you your hair looks a bit shabby, it impacts you deeply; whereas when some stranger on the street says it, you shrug it off. The voice that has the greatest impact on your cells is actually your own. Your cells respond chemically in a more pronounced way to your own voice than to the voice of anyone else, no matter how successful, brilliant and powerful that person is. Your brain takes you as the expert on everything. It will automatically respond to what you say as absolute truth. Therefore, what you speak becomes your reality. You can see then, why it is especially important to speak empowering, life-giving words that leave space for possibility.

If you are ill, every time you state: "I feel like crap," or "I'm so tired," or "My fibromyalgia..." you are affirming and recreating your state of illness. Your entire body is listening and these words are programming it what to do: create negative biochemicals that make you ill. A possibility infused statement like: "My body is processing something; I will feel so much better soon" gets your message across that something significant is going on, but puts you in an empowered state, and invites your body to receive the idea that it is doing something productive and will soon be even better. The body responds accordingly and chemical changes occur to bring about health.

Always state the positive aspect of your desire. Instead of saying: "I'd better get going because I don't want to be late for my appointment," say: "I will get going so that I arrive on time for my appointment." If you are already late, stay positive and state: "My timing is perfect and elegant and I trust that all things are in order," or "The Universe always works everything out for me, and this will work out too."

Instead of stating to your friend or child: "Be careful so you don't fall/get in an accident/trip/etc.," state: "Be careful so you stay steady/arrive safely/stay healthy/ etc." These words keep the mind centered on the desired outcome. What you focus on is what you are creating; so speak what you want to create. Children are especially vulnerable to the power of words.

When describing a frustrating situation, instead of: "My boss is a witch and always criticizes me," state: "I'm feeling frustrated with her behavior and I am inviting in more respect." Instead of: "I never get what I really want in life," state: "I would love to have more positive experiences in life than I have had in the past." This honors your frustration while inviting in a new possibility.

Avoid using "never" or other strongly negative words, or labeling things in a static way. Life is always in flux. When something seems to be stuck, it is only because you have recreated it the same way over and over and over. Make a change in how you see it. These little tweaks in how you use your words create the life you desire by keeping you in a positive and empowered place.

Life is constantly changing, and possibility abounds, so have your language reflect this and you will invite newness and joy into your life.

Thrive Tool

For the next one week, be mindful of your words. Choose to speak empowering words that reflect the life you would like to be living, in contrast to words that describe and reflect the one you are currently in. Instead of describing what you do not want in a certain situation, state what you DO want in your experience.

Question

But I am feeling ill. Does this mean I should just lie?

Lying actually generates a negative biochemistry. Speak possibility even when you are speaking about something you do not want. If you have been ill for years and are frustrated and scared that nothing will help you, a possibility statement would be: "I have been ill for years and none of the things I've tried before have helped, so I'm scared this will not work either. Sometimes I feel hopeless" instead of: "My illness is so bad that nothing ever works for me. It's hopeless." The latter affirms the situation you do not want, while the former leaves space open for possibility while still communicating your truth.

Let the new thoughts in, even if they are not yet apparent in your reality. Begin to base your thoughts and beliefs not on what you are currently experiencing, but on what you would like to be true. Choose thoughts that make you feel how you would like to feel.

Affirmation

"I speak possibility and life responds accordingly."

"Questions provide the key to unlocking our unlimited potential."

— Tony Robbins

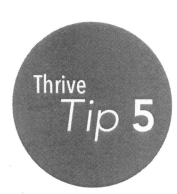

Thrive
Tip 5

Ask a Better Question

Your mind is absolutely brilliant, so why hasn't it figured out the solutions to your greatest challenges? It has never been asked to do so. The mind is constantly turning its wheels and will answer any question thrown at it. It retrieves answers the way a dog will chase and retrieve a bone. The key is to ask your mind to retrieve the kind of information that assists you in creating what you want.

With all the negative media we are faced with the mind is typically racing with worries of disaster. It asks: "What's wrong with me? Why haven't I gotten my finances together? Why isn't my lover more attentive to my needs?"

The brain delivers the answers to whatever questions you have. Therefore, your mind is filled with all the things that are wrong with you all the things that are not working in your life. Since your thoughts create your internal state, this leaves you in a perpetual negative biochemical state and causes mental and cellular impairment. Because your internal state is the basis for your external reality, this also recreates whatever challenges you are experiencing.

If you instead, center the mind on positive and

expansive questions, your brain will bring you totally different information and generate a state of inspiration. Ask yourself: "What's the best thing about me?" or "What's the best thing I could do to get the result I want?"

This tool dramatically changed my life. I had just been dumped and felt like my world was over. It was a done deal and I knew I had to accept it as it was. I asked: "How is this the best thing that could have happened for me?" Immediately I became aware of the myriad of things in the relationship that were not a fit, and I was very clear that had we stayed together, I would never have what I most wanted. It was amazing how quickly this question brought me totally different information that inspired me and made me hugely appreciative of my situation.

Our brain is hardwired to create. Neurological pathways are set in place and will deliver the same information over and over until you make changes in the programming. Asking better questions rewires your brain by causing the neurologic synapses to connect in a different way. This changes the architecture of your brain so that it thinks differently. When we think differently we create an entirely different life.

Once these new neurologic pathways are set, the mind automatically generates life-giving thoughts. Without you even trying, you generate positive emotional states that energize you and drive inspired action. Therefore, with practice, asking better questions delivers you an inspired life.

Another great way to ask better questions is to use "What if" questions to instill the positive biochemical state of Thriving and create the results you want. You don't even need answers. Just feel the response when you ask: "What if I were totally healthy and at peace?" "What if things began to come to me way more easily than I ever imagined?" "What if reading this book was the best thing I ever did?" "What if my life transforms now?" *"What if what is being said here is true and I really can receive my deepest desires?"*

Release the little voice in your head that says this is silly, this isn't working or this is too simple to be effective. Release the old, grungy way of thinking that has been dictating your life. That's just your old programming. Let go of focusing on what hasn't changed yet and try it!

Thrive Tool

Every time you find yourself challenged and you face a choice, ask: "What could I easily do now that would enhance my life the most?" If you find yourself in a negative situation you cannot change, ask: "How is this the best thing that has ever happened to me?" Then let go and let the answers come.

Question

Don't I have to figure things out? How can I get answers if I don't ask about my problem?

Your mind finds the "how" automatically for you. The information you need will come to mind. All you need to do is set your mind to your desired outcome, and life takes care of the rest. Inspirations and solutions will become apparent when you generate positive thoughts. Stop trying to figure out how, and just allow yourself to imagine. Use your questions to bring you whatever it is you want.

Affirmation

"Why am I so vibrant and alive?"
"Why am I so fulfilled and happy?"

"To the mind that is still, the whole universe surrenders."

— Lao Tzu

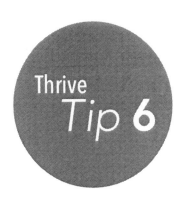

Thrive
Tip **6**

Find Your Inner Ease

The key to this tip is tuning into your emotional state and consciously bringing yourself higher. If you are feeling anxious or frustrated, whatever you do to fix the problem will not work to bring you your desired result. What you want will continue to elude you, because focusing on the problem creates the negative biochemical state that impairs your performance, clouds your judgment, and deteriorates your cells. You can't use a negative mind to create a positive situation. You first have to change your mind.

Let's say you want to lose weight and get fit. You feel frustrated with your body because you think it's too fat, too flabby, unattractive and inadequate. The negative biochemical state created by your negative thoughts increases cortisol and the stress hormones, which impairs your body's ability to burn off fat. Even if you force yourself through your workout and are able to put in a full hour, this stress state you generate with your self-criticism works against you chemically, and your body will resist losing weight.

The same occurs when you try to work harder to get a better result. When you push yourself to work even though you are tired and frustrated, the work you do will be ineffective and inefficient. The negative biochemical state of frustration impairs your brain function, making it impossible to see the big picture, come up with creative solutions and tap into insight and inspired thinking.

Often, I do my best work after taking a break to exercise or taking a nap. Things flow effortlessly and it takes me a fraction of the time to complete something I was previously struggling to complete. Always when I am frustrated and shift my internal state first, my actions and efforts work to bring about my desired result. This works for anything and anytime you are having distress. Find your inner ease by gifting yourself a hot bath, a nap, a walk, or a personal pep talk. Release guilt, fear or whatever resistance you have to doing these things. Be willing to do whatever will bring you into a more peaceful inner state.

Here's a way I recently applied this principle:

I was driving on the highway on my way to an appointment. For some reason there was tons of traffic, and I began to get that sinking feeling that comes when I know I'm going to be late. I was bummed...but I was aware! I was totally aware of feeling bummed out, thinking that I should have taken the alternative route I usually take, and that I should have left earlier. I was also wishing I were like those perfect people in my head who are always on time.

I brought my attention to my feelings of dread and anxiety, and I took a few deep breaths. I began to remember that the only important thing to do is feel good. I told myself that it would somehow be okay that I was late: maybe I wasn't meant to be on time and maybe something even better would happen. I considered that perhaps there was just an obstruction ahead and this would all clear – and I felt a bit better. I told myself that everything happens in perfect order and I remembered that things always have worked out for me, even when I didn't understand how they possibly could.

I sat in the traffic, but now was almost totally at peace. Just as this peaceful feeling began to sink in the traffic started flowing a little better and a little better and a little better, until within a minute I was up to full speed. There was no obstruction, construction or accident on the road, just sudden movement of traffic exactly at the point where I began to generate peace!

This is how the process of clearing up our internal space works to clear up our external environment. Not only was I not late as I had initially begun to anticipate, but I arrived at my appointment three minutes early! I experienced ease in my life situation because I let go of my expectation and connected with inner ease. This works like magic when you are in an argument with your spouse.

Get present, breathe, and find your inner ease in the moment no matter what is happening. Stop defending and release your resistance. You will immediately stop generating the negative biochemicals that are clouding your judgment and preventing you from seeing the big picture. You will gain insight and be able to consider the other's point of view. Often this is the exact thing that is most needed in the moment: the ability to see the other's point of view without defending yourself or accusing your spouse as wrong.

Thrive Tool

The next time you are in a negative state or you are experiencing a situation you do not want, ask yourself what it is that you most need. It may be love, rest, or physical comfort. Then imagine how it would feel to receive it.

Hold that feeling in your body for several breaths and receive it. Breathe this way until you feel an emotional shift inside.

Question

How do I feel ease when I'm feeling really really bad? When you are feeling bad, so much of your attention goes onto what you do not want and it generates more negative biochemicals. It can be challenging to break this cycle and feel better. You first have to notice that you are feeling bad. If you can bring your thoughts to what you do want or to the opposite of what's going on, that will change things up, but sometimes the problem is just too overwhelming and in our face! At these times, I simply embrace the pain. That's right, embracing and allowing is actually a positive biochemical state, even if it is pain that we are embracing! If I'm angry, I'll shout: "I'm so freaking angry!" (Sometimes just in my head.) If I'm scared, I'll just lean into how scared I really am and take a few breaths. This always dissipates the negativity and gets me to a state that feels better.

Affirmation

"I stay centered in ease, and life works out the details to support me."

*"Whatever the mind of man
can conceive and believe,
it can achieve."*

— *Napoleon Hill*

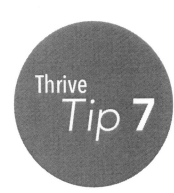

Thrive *Tip* **7**

Be Clear of Your Ultimate Outcome

Your brain is like the most brilliantly designed machine ready to serve you in any way in every moment. When you do not realize this, it's like having a Lear jet with autopilot capabilities to fly you wherever you want to go... and using it for local access as you steer it up and down the same streets manually.

The mind has access to more information than you could possibly imagine. Your expansive mind knows things from the square root of 42 to the best place for you to have dinner tonight in order to have the most fun. How do you tap into your mind's expansive capabilities? Be clear of your ultimate outcome. What exactly is it that you want in life? In a relationship? In your career? In your financial situation? What does your ideal life look like?

When you enter in your exact destination by getting clear, your mind guides you in creating it. When you get your mind clear and focused on exactly what you want, it's like setting your internal GPS to your desired destination. Your mind is constantly taking orders and creating based on what you think about. The thing is, you've been all over the place with your focus and instruction.

One minute you may think: "I want a fabulous lover and a lifelong partnership," and the next moment you think: "There are no good men out there." Maybe you think: "I would love a vacation," then you think: "I don't make enough money." Your mind delivers your experience according to the information you tell it. It will always present you with information and experiences to prove you right.

You are programming your brain on what kind of information to deliver. This is just like turning the dial on your radio and receiving different music. All of the radio waves for the different radio channels are surrounding you now. You cannot see them, but they are all there simultaneously. So it is with the information the brain is delivering to you. It depends on the way the networks in your brain are set up. You train your mind to pick up a certain frequency of information depending on what you program it to receive.

When you program your brain for the outcome you want, your neural pathways shift and your brain sets an internal map to deliver your end result. It's like a program set up to point you in the right direction in every moment.

You may be inspired to go to a certain coffee shop, where you meet exactly the person who can assist you with your business endeavor. Perhaps you suddenly think of an old friend and call him only to find that he was in need of support. When you set your mind clearly on your ultimate outcome, your inner drives will motivate you and inspire you to act and behave in ways that bring about this end result. It changes the information you notice and alters what you pay attention to.

When I wanted to create a life-partnership, I had already been through a ton of challenge in my relationships, so I decided to get completely clear on all the things I wanted in my ideal mate. This way I would clearly recognize him when he showed up in my life, and also stop fooling myself when someone was clearly not my ideal mate.

I made a list with three columns, in the left column, I listed the "must haves." These were items I would absolutely not do without. After all the relationships I'd been through, I had really come to know myself and my desires. I was clear on my absolutes and knew I fully deserved them! I listed things like compassionate, kind, loving, authentic, available, financially secure, wants to be married and have kids, and completely committed to and in love with me.

In the middle column, I listed the "it would be nice ifs." These were items I was excited about but knew would not be deal breakers if they were not there, like "has a great butt and is a fabulous skier."

In the last column listed my "absolutely nots." These were the red-flag items that I was completely clear I would not accept under any circumstances. I appreciated all of my negative experiences for teaching me this, and listed: "uses drugs, lies, smokes, spends money he doesn't have, and has no sexual boundaries."

I put the list aside and skipped about life enjoying meeting new people, because I wasn't busy thinking about whether I could make it work for the long term. I was already clear. Less than four months later I met my now-husband. He is absolutely everything I had imagined and so much more!

Thrive Tool

Create a list in an area where you desire transformation in your life. Describe your ideal ultimate outcome. Get clear on what is a "must have," "it would be nice if," and "absolutely not" for you.

Then, make a commitment to this list. Let nothing be more important to you.

Option: do this for each area of your life- relationship, career, finances, health, home, social - and commit to your desired result for each of these areas.

Question

What if I do not know the exact job I want or the specifics of what I want in life?

Even when you are not clear of the details, you can be very clear of the things that are most important to you. Let's say you want a career where you're thriving,

making plenty of money, enjoying yourself, and doing
what you are best at and love to do. Would it matter
specifically what you are doing? If there are other
factors that are important to you like, prestige, respect
and independence, add them to your list. This is your
design! It's actually helpful not to have too many
specifics, but to be totally clear on what you do know
is important.

Add to your list: "this or something even better"
to get your mind centered on the idea of greater
possibilities you can conceive of yourself. This effects
your neurology and keeps you open to greater
possibility.

Affirmation

"Life is on my side."

"I finally realized that being grateful to my body was key to giving more love to myself."

— Oprah Winfrey

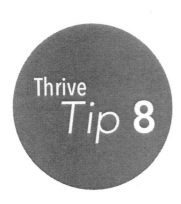

Thrive
Tip 8

Love Yourself

Love is the most powerful force in the universe. It heals illness, feeds the poor, and gets people to do outlandish things like drive for endless hours or fly across the country weekly. If you are yearning for a life of Thriving, chances are you could use more love in your life. You may imagine this love coming from outside yourself and envision an ideal lover or soul mate, who will bring this love to you, only to find yourself continually disappointed that you are not getting the love you want. Life doesn't work this way in love or in any other area of our experience. Your external life is a representation of your internal state. The love you experience, you invite in through loving yourself. When you create love by loving yourself, you are a magnet for love.

Love is also a verb, and to receive it, it's a matter of giving it – to yourself. When you love yourself, you generate positive biochemicals that make your cells Thrive. Endorphins, oxytocin, acetylcholine and antioxidants increase, making you feel energized, calm and content. This generates inspiration to behave in ways that attract others and invite connection. You therefore, experience loving relationships when you first love yourself!

Your body is the most immediate interface your thoughts have with the external world. The thoughts you have about your body create your physical form. So when you think: "Ugh, my thighs are so flabby..." or some such critical thought, your thighs are listening and will continue to form in that way. Any negative thought you have about your body will diminish the Life Force and vitality flowing to that area.

So instead, send LOVE. That's right, even to your "less-than-perfect" bum. Start with the parts of your body that are easier to appreciate. Maybe you have beautiful eyelashes, smooth cheeks, knees that bend easily, two arms to reach out and hug someone. Send love. Say: "I love you" to your symmetrical kneecaps or cute toes. Then move on to areas you currently judge to be less-than-stellar. Say hello to your wide calves in a new way. Find something you appreciate about them. I was once asked to write an ode to my thighs and it changed my relationship with them forever.

When you bring your focus to a part of your body, you actually change the chemistry in that area of the body. If you use loving, positive attention, this works to heal a sprained ankle or to generate glow in your cheeks.

When you focus your attention on an area of the body, the area in the brain that corresponds to that body part lights up with increased activity. Awareness of an injured area while feeling the emotion of love actually decreases inflammation, cellular toxicity and tissue damage. This enhances healing and restores normal function to the area.

Your loving attention to an area of your body causes the sensory receptors in that area to have enhanced sensitivity. There is more blood flow to that area which means improved nutrient and oxygen delivery and improved removal of waste products and lymphatic fluid. Inflammation clears and health is enhanced. Your body will feel better and will also function better.

When you bring negative attention to a body part, the opposite occurs. Pain sensitivity is enhanced and you propagate a pain cycle. Vascular constriction occurs and causes decreased nutrient and oxygen delivery to the cells and buildup of waste products. The pH of the tissues is decreased and muscles go into spasm. Ageing and cellular degeneration are accelerated and tissue sags and wrinkles. That is how the parts of your body that you do not like end up becoming more displeasing. Your cells are literally listening to your every thought about them and are responding accordingly. Giving your body attention in the positive state of love and appreciation makes your cells sing with vibrance and vitality.

Open yourself to receiving all kinds of love and appreciation by giving it to yourself. Whenever I catch myself looking at a part of my body with any judgment, I override all lesser thoughts by consciously saying: "I love you, I love you, I love you," until I take my attention away from it. I know negative attention will only cause discord in my body, and this can only create what I do not want. Loving myself is helping my body to heal remarkably fast from a C-section; I feel wonderful and love how I look.

Your beautiful body allows you to do so much in the world. It even digests non-food items you may be trying to feed it with. Give it a break from critical mind banter and begin to send it the appreciation it deserves.

Thrive Tool

Bring your awareness and attention to whatever area has been beat down by your judgment and mentally say: "I love you" over and over and over. Do it every time you look in the mirror. Do it any time you stop at a traffic light. Do it when you take a shower. Touch those areas and send love.

If you have an especially challenged body image or an injured body part, do this while looking in the mirror for several minutes a day. This will transform your relationship with your body, and also change how you look.

Question

How do I love something that I find unacceptable? Won't I just keep recreating that thing I don't want?

Your natural state is one of Thriving, and appreciation brings vitality to every area of your body and your life. So even if you are certain there is nothing good about the way you are, as you open to appreciation you will begin to perceive things you have not noticed before and will bring enhanced vitality to whatever your loving attention is placed upon. This will generate change in the body that pleases you.

Meditation

Visualize a warm golden light coming into your body through the top of your head and filling your entire form. Focus especially on areas where there is pain or injury and let this golden light infiltrate that area fully.

"If one advances confidently in the direction of his dreams, and endeavors to live the life which he has imagined, he will meet with a success unexpected in common hours."

— Henry David Thoreau

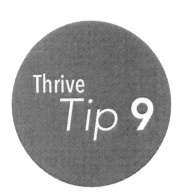

Thrive *Tip* **9**

Say "Yes" to Your YESes

Did you know people who live a life filled with
passion live approximately a decade longer, are more
successful, and have a better quality of life than those
who do not?

Your passions generate a sense of aliveness and vitality
within you that is the elixir of life and the fountain of
youth. Your passions, the things that light you up and
that you would live and die for, put you in the positive
biochemical state whether you are doing them or just
thinking about them.

According to a study at Stanford University, that
looked at people who reported to be consistently
happy, those who exhibited the greatest success all
noted that the most important thing they based their
decisions on was: passion. Not finances, not logic, not
practicality, not what others expected from them. They
made their choices based on what they were most
passionate about doing.

What if you lived life in accordance with that which
inspires you most? How would you feel getting up
every morning? What would your relationships look
like? How would your body feel? How motivated

would you be to be doing your daily life? Why aren't you making this the most important thing?

So many of the people I treat and coach are unhappy and unhealthy because they are out of alignment with this very important piece. They spend the better part of their day doing things that do not give them much (if any) energy and inspiration, and then do all kinds of things in an attempt to feel better. They are overworked, beat-down, exhausted and depressed. All the medication in the world will not make up for the depletion that comes from living your life in this way.

When you have a life without passion, you are constantly putting more energy into things than you get out of them. This means you generate more metabolic waste and toxicity than your body has the resources to manage. When you do what you are passionate about, the opposite occurs. You actually open to receiving greater amounts of energy, so you feel vitalized.

Doing what you are passionate about, or even just thinking about doing it, increases endorphins, antioxidants and oxytocin and you feel good. It also brings about changes in your neurotransmitters that opens you to information and awareness than you would not otherwise have. You are more efficient and effective, more intuitive, and guided to do the actions that are needed to generate your desired result.

The way you structure your life is entirely up to you, and what you prioritize will be what gets most of your energy and attention. The most important thing you can do is to order your life in alignment with the things that are most important to you; the things you care about and would give your life for. That is what you are doing; giving your life: time energy, effort and attention. Be willing and committed to give your life to your passions, and your body will reap the rewards.

How do you identify your passions? Your passions may be things like "feeling healthy and fit" or "spending quality time with my family" or "enjoying wealth and prosperity." Your passion is anything that makes your heart sing.

I call choosing your passions "Saying 'Yes' to Your YESes." In our Unleashing the Physician Within course, I emphatically teach that our inner drives and deepest yearnings are the ignition to our greatest success. It is our inner YES that points us in the direction of inspiration. In your natural state of Thriving, you follow this feeling and choose the choice that resonates with it. This means if you're trying to complete some work and are not getting anywhere, but are yearning for a hot bath, a long walk, a nap, or a break with a friend – TAKE IT!

Your inner YES is not ambiguous. It's the "OH YAY!" feeling you initially get when you consider something that sounds really good. It may not last long because it is often followed by a: "Yeah, but...(fill in the limiting, fear-based belief that drowns out your inner YES)". The fear-based belief may look like: "That would never work out," or "Who the heck am I to think I can do THAT?" or "That is ridiculous!" The limiting thought may even try to confuse you with doubt by saying: "I don't really know what I want." You DO! It just jumped out as a feeling of vast excitement that looked completely ridiculous and irrational! That's your passion calling!

Research at Stanford University has shown that true happiness and thriving comes not from following the "rules" as you have been taught: study hard, get a good job, work your tail off and you'll be all set. Not only will you clearly not be "all set" but you won't even be remotely okay. Most people trying to retire today have had to add another decade or so to their work–days. Most people who follow this prescription do not enjoy what they do, and suffer immense health consequences. Even if financial abundance follows, the misery associated with a life devoid of passion leads to expensive addictions, expensive medical bills and expensive divorces! People who follow these "rules" are miserable. None of the highly successful people I've ever studied, or who were cited in the above study lived life according to this traditional model.

What creates a life of thriving is being true to you. Your inner YES guides you there. Listen every day and be willing to follow and say: "yes" to your YES! It is your aliveness and your ticket to thriving! Your YES is your internal GPS that guides you to your thriving life.

Follow your passion and choose what most deeply serves you. Every time you have a choice of any kind, ask yourself, what am I most excited about? Feel for your inner YES and follow it. Know that you are free to make any choice you desire. Make passion-based choices and create a life that sustains you, where you get to be who you really are, live your truth and express your authentic self. This always leads to the rejuvenation, inspiration, chance meetings or a totally new path that is the fastest road to your success.

Thrive Tool

Ask yourself: "Now that I am living my ideal life, I am _____." Fill in the blank with actions you would be doing if you were in your ideal life. Distill this list down to your top five and write them on index cards. Place them where you will be reminded several times daily. This keeps your attention on your passions and brings them into your life.

Question

How can I just do what I want all the time? Don't I need to compromise and serve others in order to make life work?

Compromise will never make your life work. You are in the driver's seat, and every time you compromise yourself, you buy into something that will not serve you and generates the negative biochemical state. The urge to compromise comes from a fear-based belief that who you are exactly as you are is not enough. This is a negative thought and is therefore, life-depleting. The Truth is, you can have the life you desire just for being you. Honoring your own unique passions is the greatest service you can do for everyone you care about.

When you are in the inspired state of passion, you actually have greater awareness of the unity of all people and have more compassion, understanding and love for others. Living your passion is your greatest gift to the world.

Affirmation

"When faced with a choice, I choose in favor of my passions!"

"If we could change ourselves, the tendencies in the world would also change. As a man changes his own nature, so does the attitude of the world change towards him."

— Mahatma Gandhi

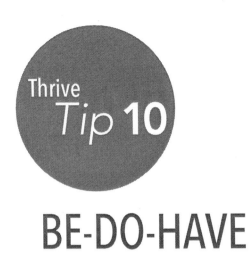

Thrive *Tip* **10**

BE-DO-HAVE

I've come across this formula in multiple courses, books and teachings on success, either spelled out or implied. It is the no-fail, tried and true, secret to success that all masters use and most people get completely backwards. I have applied it to my own life and it always works. I've attracted work I love, friends I adore, an amazing life-partner and family of my own, and beautiful places to live every time I've desired to move.

I've done this by learning how to BE that which I desire to be, even when my external life does not reflect or support that. The first part of the equation is the most important. BEing happy or anything else, can only happen now and can only happen when you choose it.

What actually works unfailingly in attracting your heart's desire is: BE-DO- HAVE. Once you are able to BE happy, you shift immediately into the positive biochemical state. This state drives all of your actions and behaviors. You have inspiration and vitality so you can sustain your work and your workout! Your brain works better so everything occurs to you differently. The things you are inspired and energized to DO will be actions and behaviors that create the kinds of things that support your positive emotional state. You then HAVE that which supports your positive state of BEing. These actions and behaviors are easy to maintain, because your state of BEing supports them. Life becomes effortless, and having what you want is an inevitable result.

You've been taught that the key to happiness and success is to attain or achieve a certain thing, and once you HAVE that, you will be able to DO what you want, and then you will BE happy. The thing you want may be a nice house, a job, an amount of money, a marriage, children, your ideal body weight...and you may be completely convinced that once you have attained this thing you will then be fulfilled. You can't even imagine being happy and fulfilled without these things being met. Maybe you do not feel worthy of just BEing happy now. Maybe you do not feel you have done enough to deserve that. Perhaps you don't even believe it's possible to just BE happy without having achieved or attained these items first.

All of these are just beliefs. Even if they are based on your experiences, they are still just beliefs. These experiences have you convinced that you absolutely need to first HAVE a certain thing in order to BE happy. You may be so convinced of this, you work in a job you don't enjoy, hold off on dating someone you're really psyched about, or spend years pursuing goals that are not your true passions.

When you focus on the HAVE and then DO what you think you should be doing in order to get to BE what you want, you are not living in a state of vitality and aliveness. Let's say you want to have a nice home with your happy family. You've been taught to get a good job so you can pay for the home, and that you need an education so that you can get a good job. What you really want to do is create art, or travel around the world, but instead you go to school. You do this because you think it will bring you all of these things you want, even though your heart isn't in it. You live in a negative biochemical state because you are doing something you do not really want to do. Life is empty. Because you are empty and without real aliveness, no one hires you. You don't create an inspired life because you are not inspired.

Life doesn't work this way because when your inspiration is missing, it's just an empty life. That's why even when you get all of the things you think you need to HAVE, you are ultimately unfulfilled. All the beautiful homes in the world will not bring you what you are looking for.

When you go after having things because you think
they will bring you a desired end result, there is
no passion to drive your actions. When you do life
according to: HAVE-DO-BE, it never works to generate
true fulfillment and thriving. Never.

Why is it impossible? There are three reasons this will
never work. One is that you can never experience
happiness, peace or true fulfillment when you base it
in the future. Happiness can only exist now, because
life occurs in the present.

The second reason is that as long as you make your
happiness contingent on having something external,
whether that is an item, an achievement, or a number
on the scale, it is conditional, and it will always be
linked to the fear of losing that thing. True happiness,
peace, or thriving is generated within, is unconditional,
and cannot be taken away.

The third reason this approach does not work is
because your life always reflects your internal state.
When you go after things you are not truly passionate
about just because you think that once you attain
them they will bring you happiness, you are not in the
positive biochemical state. Unless what you are DOing

is derived out of BEing in the state of joy, passion and appreciation, they will not bring you reasons to experience more joy, passion or appreciation. The joy and happiness that come from attaining a goal are limited and fleeting unless they are derived from a state of first BEing joyful and happy. When you are first BEing happy (or successful, fulfilled, worthy,) all the circumstances to support it come flooding into your life. They can't not come into your experience.

So how do you get into an inspired state of BEing? Imagine what you desire (a slim fit body, money, success, freedom, partnership...) and feel what it would be like to have that now. Feel how it feels to live that experience. You will begin to generate endorphins, oxytocin, antioxidants, and other positive biochemicals. You also shift your brain into an expansive, winning mindset. This gives you energy, motivation and inspiration to take the actions that bring about your desired outcome.

The next step is: DO. What would you be doing if you were a huge success? What choices would you make? How would you stand, walk, speak? How would you move if you were loved beyond measure? What would you look like if you were happy now? Your physiologic state is deeply dependent on your posture and your motions. Even just how you stand creates your internal state! Standing in a slumped position with shoulders hunched and head hanging low makes it impossible to harbor joyful, happy, vibrant thoughts. In contrast, standing erect, shoulders back and head held high makes it inevitable that you hold thoughts of empowerment, strength and joy. Even the simple act of smiling induces a state of happiness by increasing hormones that initiate this state. So DO whatever it is you are inspired to do if you from that state of BEing that you are wanting to BE. Do what feels natural from this state of BEing.

When you are BEing in your desired state, the DOing comes easily as a result of this. You don't have to think about it or try. Your state of BEing is evident in your voice: your tone, volume, pace, even your pauses. All of these convey your success, and affect everyone around you.

From this heightened state of existence you will HAVE the life circumstances consistent with staying in that state. Because your DOing stems from a heightened state of BEing, you create an effect that supports you. People treat you differently, new opportunities open up to you, and relationships are smooth and connected. Your physiology responds positively so you will create a more fit healthy body. Put your energy and attention on the BE, and HAVEing is effortless.

Thrive Tool

Act as if. Stand as if you were a great success. Walk and move as if you were deeply loved and cherished. Speak as if you had great security and deep peace. It is through BEing that which you are desiring to BE, that you create a life that supports you in being this.

Hold that feeling in your body for several breaths and receive it. Breathe this way until you feel an emotional shift inside.

Question

If I just decide to be happy now, exactly as I am, won't I lose all motivation to make a change? It's not really okay for me to stay exactly as I am.

It may take a little faith at first to see if this works. Maybe for years you've been told to work hard to HAVE security, and once you have it, then you can DO what you really want to do. Maybe you believe that you will finally BE happy once you meet a romantic partner. Release your ideas about how life works. You have been running a rat race. Security, peace, love or any other state you desire comes from within and is available to you now. Try it and look for evidence of your life responding.

Affirmation

"I am safe and secure in the power of my own inner knowing."

Conclusion

We live in a world where information and new ideas
are transmitted instantly and things are moving
forward so quickly in the evolution of the human race.
In the past, it took decades for our culture to embrace
new ideas and assimilate a new belief into our way of
doing things. The idea that women are equal to men
was at first laughed at, then ridiculed, then fought
against violently, until finally it was integrated fully and
society continued as if this had always been the case
with an attitude that "of course it is so."

This new idea I've presented, that our internal state is
the premise for our external reality, is also in a process
of integration. This idea was initially shunned, then
adamantly fought and is now being embraced by
millions. You will be somewhere along the continuum
of this process as you too integrate this new
understanding.

It is my intention that our society will release old fears
and old ways of being, so that we embrace this deeper

understanding of reality and fully integrate it into our systems of education and healthcare. This societal change begins with each of us individually. Your impact is far greater than you can imagine. Use these tools to assist you in coming to your own realization of this Truth.

Anything you desire to change in the world is within your capability of changing. The change begins within you. It does not come about by manipulating your situation or fighting against things that bother you or that you disagree with. The change comes when you embrace your frustration with the world as your own internal state. Choose to shift this frustration within yourself. When you shift yourself, the world shifts. This is the way we create a reality where everyone wins.

Quantum Physics shows us that there is nothing outside us that is not impacted by our observation of it. If I feel sad for starving children in Africa, it is sadness to be cleared within me. If I feel angry about abused animals, that anger is my internal pollution. When I take responsibility for my own negative states I am empowered to do what needs to be done to generate real change in the world. This empowerment changes the way my words are heard and the impact they have. This empowerment enables me to inspire others to behave in ways that are consistent with respecting our world. This empowerment creates a space of clarity wherein we all see Truth.

I invite you to apply these Thrive Tips and do whatever is needed to empower yourself so that you are awake and inspired and can assist in creating a beautiful world for yourself and for us all! Choose your favorites and share them.

Together, we thrive!

About the Author

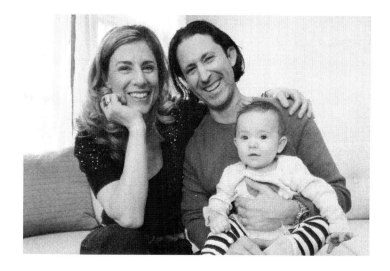

Dr. Kimberly D'Eramo is a board-certified emergency medicine physician trained in osteopathic manipulative medicine, who has been practicing Thrive-based medicine for over a decade. Throughout her practice, she has come to understand the Universal Principles that make us Thrive and make life work.

In applying these principles to her own life, Dr. D'Eramo has experienced miraculous results – from reversing chronic illness to meeting her life partner and creating a successful business. She unites these Universal Principles to the practice of medicine so that we may apply medical treatment and procedures in a way that works consistently. This combination maximizes the potential of our medical technologies and practitioners.

Together with her husband, Dr. Mario Torres-Leon, Dr. D'Eramo co-founded The Thrive Doctors: teaching the science behind how we heal, so you can consciously create your health and your life. Visit them at: www. thethrivedoctors.com for further resources, and to join their Thrive Movement.

In addition to being a physician and author, she is also a professional speaker, coach and entrepreneur. Dr. D'Eramo currently practices osteopathic medicine in the Boston area, where she lives with her husband and their daughter Gemma.